Menopause Madness: A Hilarious Guide to Figuring it Out

Table of Contents:

1. **Welcome to the Rollercoaster Ride:** Introducing Menopause and Its Wild Adventures
2. **The Hormonal Highway:** Navigating Mood Swings and Hot Flashes
3. **The Battle of the Bulge:** Conquering Weight Gain and Metabolism Mayhem
4. **Sleepless in Menopause:** Surviving Nights of Sweats and Insomnia
5. **The Memory Maze:** Losing Your Keys and Your Mind, But Finding Humor Along the Way
6. **The Vaginal Chronicles:** From Dryness to Discomfort, a Comedy of Errors
7. **The Joy of Joints:** Embracing Aches and Pains with a Sense of Humor
8. **The Fashion Fiasco:** Dressing for Your Personal Tropical Climate
9. **The Libido Limbo:** Navigating the Ups and Downs of Desire
10. **The Partner Predicament:** Explaining Menopause to Your Significant Other Without Starting World War III
11. **The Beauty Buffet:** Embracing Your Inner Goddess Despite the Wrinkles and Gray Hairs

12. **Menopause, Mastery, and Mayhem:** Finding Peace, Laughter, and Sanity in the Midst of Hormonal Chaos

Chapter 1: Welcome to the Rollercoaster Ride

Welcome aboard the tumultuous journey of menopause – a rollercoaster of hormonal havoc that promises thrills, spills, and more twists and turns than a soap opera plot. As you strap in for the wild ride ahead, prepare to experience the highs and lows of this hormonal highway without a roadmap in sight.

Picture yourself standing at the threshold of an amusement park, staring down the tracks of a colossal coaster that taunts with its loops and dips. This isn't just any theme park attraction – it's the ride of your life, and you're about to buckle up for the wildest adventure yet.

As the coaster clanks to life and begins its ascent, anticipation mounts like the first inklings of a hot flash. You're about to dive headfirst into the tempest of menopause, where mood swings reign supreme and hot flashes are the fiery dragons you never knew you feared.

Let's start with mood swings – the emotional rollercoaster that threatens to derail even the most stoic of passengers. One moment, you're laughing uproariously at a cat video, and the next, you're sobbing into your pillow because the cat reminded you of your childhood pet. It's a whirlwind of emotions that leaves you feeling like you're navigating a minefield blindfolded.

But fear not, for mood swings are just one of the many attractions on this hormonal thrill ride. Think of them as the unexpected detours that add spice to an otherwise mundane journey. From inexplicable rage over burnt toast to uncontrollable fits of laughter during a serious conversation, every mood swing is a reminder that you're alive and kicking – even if it feels like your emotions are kicking you in the gut.

Now, let's talk about hot flashes – the fiery eruptions that turn your body into a personal sauna at the most inconvenient times. Picture this: you're in the middle of a boardroom presentation, charming potential clients with your wit and wisdom, when suddenly, you feel it – a wave of heat washing over you like a tsunami. Your cheeks flush, your palms sweat, and all you can think about is stripping off your clothes and diving into the nearest ice bath.

But here's the kicker: hot flashes are the great equalizer of menopause. They don't care if you're a CEO or a stay-at-home mom, a supermodel or a soccer coach – when the heat hits, you're all in the same sweaty boat. So why not embrace the madness and invest in a stylish collection of handheld fans? Trust me, nothing says "I'm a force to be reckoned with" quite like a fan bedazzled with rhinestones and glitter.

As the coaster hurtles through another hair-raising turn, you cling to the safety bar with white-knuckled determination, wondering what other surprises menopause has in store for you. But amidst the chaos and confusion, there's a sense of camaraderie that comes from knowing you're not alone on this wild ride. Whether you're commiserating with coworkers over shared hot flash horror stories or swapping mood swing anecdotes with friends over cocktails, there's comfort in knowing that you're all in this together.

So buckle up, buttercup, and get ready for the ride of your life. Menopause may be a rollercoaster of epic proportions, but with a healthy dose of humor and a supportive network of fellow riders, you'll make it through with your sanity – and your sense of adventure – intact. After all, life is too short to take it too seriously, especially when you're careening through the twists and turns of menopause madness.

Chapter 2: The Hormonal Highway

Welcome to the hormonal highway, where the road signs are written in mood swings and the scenery changes faster than you can say "hot flash." As you navigate this tumultuous terrain, prepare to encounter twists, turns, and detours that will leave you feeling like you're on a never-ending journey through the depths of your own body.

Let's start with the basics: hormones. Those elusive little chemicals that have the power to make or break your day with the flick of a switch. During menopause, your hormone levels go haywire, fluctuating like a yo-yo on a caffeine bender. Estrogen, progesterone, testosterone – they all dance around each other in a delicate balancing act that's as precarious as it is unpredictable.

First up on our tour of the hormonal highway: mood swings. Ah, yes, the emotional rollercoaster that threatens to derail your sanity at every turn. One minute, you're as giddy as a schoolgirl on prom night, and the next, you're ready to unleash your inner Hulk on anyone who dares to look at you the wrong way.

But here's the thing about mood swings — they're not just random outbursts of emotion. They're the result of a hormonal cocktail that's been shaken, stirred, and served up with a side of chaos. When your estrogen levels plummet and your progesterone levels go on a rollercoaster ride of their own, it's no wonder you feel like you're teetering on the edge of a meltdown.

Next stop on our journey: hot flashes. Oh, the joys of feeling like you're spontaneously combusting in the middle of a business meeting or a romantic dinner date. It's like your body's way of saying, "Hey, remember me? I'm still here, and I'm going to make your life a living hell for the foreseeable future."

But here's the thing about hot flashes — they're not just about feeling hot and sweaty. They're a symphony of sensations that can leave you feeling dizzy, nauseous, and more than a little disoriented. From the sudden surge of heat that starts in your chest and radiates outwards like a raging inferno to the clammy aftermath that leaves you feeling like you've just run a marathon in a sauna, hot flashes are a force to be reckoned with.

But fear not, intrepid traveler, for there are ways to tame the fiery beast that is the hot flash. From dressing in layers so you can strip down at a moment's notice to investing in a portable fan that fits discreetly in your purse, there are plenty of strategies for keeping cool when the heat is on.

As the hormonal highway stretches out before you, dotted with mood swings and hot flashes like potholes in the pavement, remember this: you're not alone. Every woman who has ever embarked on this journey has encountered the same bumps in the road, the same twists and turns that make menopause feel like a never-ending rollercoaster ride.

So buckle up, my friend, and hold on tight. The hormonal highway may be a wild and unpredictable ride, but with a sense of humor and a supportive network of fellow travelers by your side, you'll make it through with your sanity – and your sense of adventure – intact. After all, life is too short to let a few hormone-induced mood swings and hot flashes derail your journey. So embrace the madness, embrace the chaos, and remember: this too shall pass.

Chapter 3: The Battle of the Bulge

Welcome to the battleground of menopausal weight gain – where the battle of the bulge takes on a whole new meaning, and the enemy seems to lurk around every corner, armed with calorie-laden treats and sedentary temptations. As you lace up your metaphorical combat boots and prepare to face this formidable foe, know that you're not alone in the fight.

First things first, let's talk about why menopause seems to have declared war on your waistline. Blame it on those pesky hormones – estrogen, progesterone, and their mischievous accomplices. As your hormone levels fluctuate and your metabolism slows to a crawl, your body becomes a battleground where calories are the enemy and fat cells are the foot soldiers.

But here's the thing about menopausal weight gain – it's not just about the number on the scale. It's about how you feel in your own skin, how your clothes fit, and how your self-esteem takes a hit every time you catch a glimpse of yourself in the mirror. It's about the frustration of trying to zip up your favorite pair of jeans and realizing they're suddenly two sizes too small. It's about the guilt and shame that come with indulging in a second helping of dessert, knowing full well that it's only going to make matters worse.

But fear not, brave warrior, for there are strategies for conquering the bulge and reclaiming your body as your own. It starts with embracing a healthy lifestyle that includes regular exercise, mindful eating, and plenty of self-care. Sure, it's not easy – especially when every fiber of your being is screaming for chocolate cake – but it's worth it in the end.

Let's start with exercise – the secret weapon in the battle of the bulge. Not only does regular physical activity help burn calories and build muscle, but it also boosts your mood and improves your overall sense of well-being. Whether you prefer yoga, swimming, or good old-fashioned cardio, find an activity that brings you joy and stick with it. Remember, exercise isn't just about losing weight – it's about feeling strong, confident, and empowered in your own body.

Next up, let's talk about mindful eating – the art of nourishing your body without depriving yourself of the foods you love. Instead of viewing food as the enemy, embrace it as fuel for your body and soul. Focus on eating whole, nutrient-rich foods that leave you feeling satisfied and energized, and indulge in treats in moderation. Remember, it's not about perfection – it's about finding balance and listening to your body's hunger and fullness cues.

And finally, let's talk about self-care — the secret weapon in your arsenal against stress, anxiety, and emotional eating. Whether it's taking a bubble bath, getting a massage, or simply taking a few deep breaths to center yourself, prioritize self-care as an essential part of your daily routine. After all, you can't pour from an empty cup, and taking care of yourself is the first step towards reclaiming your body and your life.

As the battle of the bulge rages on, remember this: you are more than a number on the scale, more than the size of your jeans, more than the sum of your parts. You are a warrior, a survivor, a force to be reckoned with — and you have the power to conquer anything that stands in your way.

So lace up those combat boots, my friend, and march boldly into battle. With a sense of determination, a healthy dose of self-love, and a supportive network of fellow warriors by your side, you'll emerge victorious in the battle of the bulge. And when you do, you'll stand tall and proud, knowing that you've reclaimed your body and your life as your own.

Chapter 4: Sleepless in Menopause

Welcome to the land of restless nights and weary mornings – where sleep is as elusive as a unicorn and insomnia reigns supreme. As you toss and turn in the darkness, your mind racing a mile a minute, know that you're not alone in the battle against sleepless nights.

Let's start with the basics: why does menopause wreak havoc on your sleep patterns? Blame it on those pesky hormones once again. As estrogen levels decline and progesterone levels fluctuate, your body's internal clock goes haywire, leaving you feeling like a zombie stumbling through the fog of exhaustion.

But here's the thing about menopausal insomnia – it's not just about tossing and turning all night. It's about the frustration of lying awake in bed, watching the minutes tick by on the clock, knowing that tomorrow's responsibilities loom large on the horizon. It's about the anxiety that creeps in as the night wears on, whispering doubts and fears into the darkness. It's about the sheer exhaustion of facing another day on an empty tank of sleep.

But fear not, weary traveler, for there are strategies for reclaiming your nights and banishing insomnia once and for all. It starts with creating a sleep-friendly environment that encourages relaxation and tranquility. From investing in a comfortable mattress and pillows to creating a calming bedtime routine, there are plenty of ways to set the stage for a restful night's sleep.

Let's start with your sleep environment – the foundation upon which restful slumber is built. Make sure your bedroom is cool, dark, and quiet, free from distractions that might disrupt your sleep. Invest in blackout curtains to block out streetlights and early morning sunlight, and consider using a white noise machine or earplugs to drown out any ambient noise that might disturb your rest.

Next, let's talk about your bedtime routine – the rituals that signal to your body that it's time to wind down and prepare for sleep. Whether it's taking a warm bath, practicing relaxation techniques like deep breathing or meditation, or simply curling up with a good book, find activities that help you unwind and relax before bed. And whatever you do, avoid stimulating activities like watching TV or scrolling through your phone in the hour leading up to bedtime – the blue light emitted by screens can interfere with your body's natural sleep-wake cycle and make it harder to fall asleep.

But what about those nights when sleep seems like an impossible dream, no matter how hard you try? That's where cognitive behavioral therapy for insomnia (CBT-I) comes in. This evidence-based treatment focuses on changing the thoughts and behaviors that contribute to insomnia, helping you develop healthy sleep habits and overcome the obstacles standing in the way of restful slumber.

As the battle against insomnia rages on, remember this: you are not powerless in the face of sleepless nights. With a combination of lifestyle changes, relaxation techniques, and, if necessary, professional guidance, you can reclaim your nights and banish insomnia once and for all.

So dim the lights, slip into your comfiest pajamas, and prepare to embrace the sweet embrace of sleep. With patience, persistence, and a healthy dose of self-care, you'll emerge from the darkness of insomnia into the light of restful slumber. And when you do, you'll awaken feeling refreshed, rejuvenated, and ready to face whatever the day may bring.

Chapter 5: The Memory Maze

Welcome to the labyrinth of forgetfulness, where memories vanish like socks in the dryer and names slip through the cracks of your mind like water through a sieve. As you navigate the twists and turns of the memory maze, know that you're not alone in the struggle against forgetfulness.

Let's start with the basics: why does menopause seem to have a knack for playing tricks on your memory? Blame it on those pesky hormones once again. As estrogen levels decline and progesterone levels fluctuate, your brain's chemistry undergoes a major overhaul, leaving you feeling like you've misplaced the key to your own mind.

But here's the thing about menopausal memory loss – it's not just about forgetting where you left your keys or blanking on your coworker's name at the office party. It's about the frustration of losing track of conversations mid-sentence, the embarrassment of forgetting important dates and appointments, and the fear that you're losing your grip on reality.

But fear not, intrepid explorer of the memory maze, for there are strategies for sharpening your mental acuity and reclaiming control of your cognitive faculties. It starts with exercising your brain like a muscle, keeping it sharp and agile through regular mental workouts and cognitive challenges.

Let's start with brain exercises – the mental equivalent of hitting the gym to pump iron and build muscle. Whether it's solving crossword puzzles, playing brain-training games on your phone, or learning a new language or skill, find activities that challenge your mind and keep your synapses firing on all cylinders. And don't forget to mix it up – variety is the spice of life, and keeping your brain engaged with a diverse range of activities will help stave off boredom and keep your mind sharp.

Next, let's talk about lifestyle factors that can impact memory and cognitive function. From getting regular exercise and eating a healthy diet to managing stress and getting enough sleep, there are plenty of lifestyle habits that can either support or sabotage your brain health. So make sure you're taking care of yourself both physically and mentally – after all, a healthy body is the foundation of a healthy mind.

keep you cool and dry, and choose colors and patterns that are forgiving of the occasional sweat stain. And remember, a sense of humor is your best accessory – because sometimes, the only way to survive a fashion fiasco is to laugh your way through it.

But dressing for your personal tropical climate isn't just about staying cool and comfortable – it's also about expressing yourself and embracing your unique sense of style. Menopause may throw some curveballs your way, but it doesn't have to cramp your fashion game. Experiment with bold colors, playful patterns, and statement accessories that reflect your personality and make you feel fabulous. After all, confidence is the best outfit you can wear – and with a little creativity and a whole lot of attitude, you can rock any look, no matter what the thermostat says.

As you navigate the fashion fiasco of menopause, remember this: you are a fierce, fabulous, and fashionable woman, capable of conquering any challenge that comes your way – even if it's just finding the perfect outfit for your personal tropical climate. So embrace the sweat stains, laugh off the wardrobe malfunctions, and strut your stuff with confidence and style. Menopause may be a fashion fiasco, but with a little humor and a lot of flair, you can turn even the sweatiest of situations into a fashion moment to remember.

Chapter 9-The Libido Limbo: Navigating the Ups and Downs of Desire

But what about those moments when your memory fails you despite your best efforts? That's where mnemonic devices and memory aids come in. Whether it's setting reminders on your phone, using sticky notes to jog your memory, or creating mnemonic devices to help you remember important information, there are plenty of tricks you can use to compensate for forgetfulness and keep your memory on track.

As you navigate the twists and turns of the memory maze, remember this: you are not defined by your forgetfulness. Memory lapses are a natural part of the aging process, and while they can be frustrating, they don't diminish your worth or your intelligence. So be kind to yourself, be patient with yourself, and remember that you're doing the best you can in a world that sometimes feels like it's slipping through your fingers.

So grab your mental map and your compass, my friend, and prepare to navigate the memory maze with confidence and resilience. With a combination of brain exercises, healthy lifestyle habits, and a healthy dose of self-compassion, you'll emerge from the labyrinth of forgetfulness stronger, wiser, and more resilient than ever before. And when you do, you'll find that the memories you cherish most are the ones that were worth the struggle to hold onto.

Chapter 6: The Vaginal Chronicles

Welcome to the intimate world of menopausal changes, where the delicate ecosystem of your nether regions undergoes a transformation that can feel like a rollercoaster ride without a seatbelt. As you journey through the twists and turns of the vaginal chronicles, know that you're not alone in grappling with the challenges and surprises that menopause can bring to this most intimate part of your body.

Let's start with the basics: why does menopause wreak havoc on your vagina? Blame it on – you guessed it – those pesky hormones. As estrogen levels decline during menopause, the tissues of your vagina become thinner, drier, and less elastic, leading to a host of uncomfortable symptoms that can range from mild irritation to downright agony.

But here's the thing about menopausal vaginal changes – they're not just about physical discomfort. They're about the impact they can have on your sexual health, your relationships, and your sense of self. From painful intercourse and chronic dryness to increased vulnerability to infections and urinary issues, the symptoms of menopausal vaginal changes can take a toll on every aspect of your life.

But fear not, brave explorer of the vaginal chronicles, for there are strategies for managing the symptoms and reclaiming your comfort and confidence. It starts with understanding your body and its changing needs, and being proactive about seeking out solutions that work for you.

Let's start with lubrication – the secret weapon in the battle against vaginal dryness. Whether it's a water-based lubricant for solo play or a silicone-based lubricant for partnered activities, finding the right lubricant can make all the difference in the world when it comes to easing discomfort and enhancing pleasure. And don't be afraid to experiment – there are plenty of different types and formulations available, so don't settle for anything less than perfect for you.

Next, let's talk about vaginal moisturizers – a must-have for menopausal women dealing with chronic dryness. Unlike lubricants, which are designed for temporary relief during sexual activity, vaginal moisturizers are formulated to hydrate and nourish the tissues of the vagina on a long-term basis. Think of them as a skincare regimen for your lady parts – something you apply regularly to keep everything feeling soft, supple, and comfortable.

But what about those pesky urinary symptoms that seem to go hand in hand with menopausal vaginal changes? That's where pelvic floor exercises come in. By strengthening the muscles of your pelvic floor, you can improve bladder control, reduce the risk of urinary incontinence, and even enhance sexual pleasure. So don't be shy about squeezing in a few Kegels throughout the day – your bladder will thank you for it.

As you navigate the twists and turns of the vaginal chronicles, remember this: you are not alone in your struggles, and there are resources available to help you navigate this intimate journey with confidence and grace. Whether it's talking to your healthcare provider about treatment options, seeking out support groups for menopausal women, or simply sharing your experiences with trusted friends and loved ones, know that you have a community of fellow travelers who understand what you're going through.

So embrace the changes, my friend, and remember that menopause is just another chapter in the ongoing saga of womanhood. With a combination of knowledge, self-care, and a healthy dose of humor, you'll emerge from the vaginal chronicles stronger, wiser, and more in tune with your body than ever before. And when you do, you'll find that the journey was worth every bump in the road – because it led you to a place of greater comfort, confidence, and self-love.

Chapter 7: The Joy of Joints

Welcome to the Joy of Joints, where creaks, cracks, and pops are the soundtrack of your everyday life. As you navigate the twists and turns of menopause, you may find yourself grappling with aches and pains that seem to come out of nowhere. But fear not, dear reader, for you are not alone in the battle against joint discomfort.

Let's start with the basics: why do your joints suddenly feel like they belong to someone twice your age? Blame it on – you guessed it – those pesky hormones. As estrogen levels decline during menopause, your body's natural anti-inflammatory response is thrown out of whack, leaving you more vulnerable to aches, pains, and stiffness.

But here's the thing about joint pain – it's not just about physical discomfort. It's about the impact it can have on your quality of life, your mobility, and your independence. From struggling to climb stairs or open jars to feeling like you're walking on eggshells with every step, joint pain can make even the simplest tasks feel like Herculean feats.

But fear not, intrepid explorer of the Joy of Joints, for there are strategies for managing the symptoms and reclaiming your comfort and mobility. It starts with understanding the root causes of your joint pain and taking proactive steps to address them.

Let's start with lifestyle factors that can exacerbate joint pain. From carrying excess weight to leading a sedentary lifestyle, there are plenty of habits that can put added strain on your joints and make your symptoms worse. So take a good look at your daily habits and see if there are any changes you can make to support your joint health. Whether it's losing weight, incorporating regular exercise into your routine, or making time for relaxation and stress relief, every little bit helps when it comes to managing joint pain.

Next, let's talk about the importance of staying active – even when your joints are screaming for mercy. Contrary to popular belief, exercise is one of the best things you can do for joint pain. Not only does it help strengthen the muscles around your joints and improve flexibility, but it also releases endorphins – your body's natural painkillers – which can help alleviate discomfort and improve your overall sense of well-being. So don't let joint pain keep you on the sidelines. Find activities that you enjoy and that are gentle on your joints, like swimming, yoga, or walking, and make them a regular part of your routine.

But what about those days when joint pain seems to be calling the shots, no matter what you do? That's where self-care comes in. Whether it's taking a warm bath, applying a soothing topical cream, or practicing relaxation techniques like deep breathing or meditation, find ways to pamper your joints and give them the TLC they deserve. And don't forget to listen to your body – if something doesn't feel right, don't push through the pain. Take a break, give yourself permission to rest, and come back to your activities when you're feeling more comfortable.

As you navigate the twists and turns of the Joy of Joints, remember this: you are not defined by your pain, and you are not alone in your struggles. With a combination of lifestyle changes, exercise, and self-care, you can manage your symptoms and reclaim your comfort and mobility. So embrace the journey, my friend, and remember that every step you take is a victory in the battle against joint pain.

Chapter 8: The Fashion Fiasco: Dressing for Your Personal Tropical Climate

Welcome to the chapter on fashion in our menopause journey – or as I like to call it, "The Fashion Fiasco: Dressing for Your Personal Tropical Climate." As we navigate the wild and unpredictable world of menopause, one thing becomes abundantly clear: dressing for this personal tropical climate is no easy feat. From hot flashes to night sweats, our bodies are like walking thermometers, constantly fluctuating between Arctic chills and Sahara heatwaves. But fear not, dear reader, for with a little creativity, a touch of humor, and a healthy dose of self-acceptance, we can conquer even the most fashionably-challenged moments of menopause.

Let's start with the basics: the hot flash – that sudden surge of heat that turns your body into a veritable furnace at the most inconvenient times. Whether you're in the middle of a business meeting, a romantic dinner, or a crowded subway car, there's no escaping the fiery inferno that rages within. So how do you dress for a personal tropical climate that can strike at any moment? The key is layers – lots and lots of layers. Think of yourself as a walking onion, with each layer providing a barrier against the heat and a quick escape route when the temperature rises. And don't forget the fan – because nothing says fashion-forward like a handheld fan in one hand and a glass of ice water in the other.

But what about those pesky night sweats – the nocturnal cousins of hot flashes that turn your bed into a swampy oasis of damp sheets and twisted covers? Dressing for bedtime can feel like a game of Russian roulette, with each pajama choice carrying the risk of waking up in a pool of your own sweat. So how do you stay cool and comfortable while you sleep? Opt for lightweight, breathable fabrics like cotton or bamboo, and choose loose-fitting styles that allow for maximum airflow. And don't be afraid to ditch the pajamas altogether – because sometimes, the only thing standing between you and a good night's sleep is the freedom to let it all hang out.

Now, let's talk about the fashion faux pas that can arise when you're dressing for your personal tropical climate. From the dreaded "sweat stains" to the unfortunate "wardrobe malfunctions," menopause can throw a wrench in even the most carefully curated outfit. But fear not, fashionistas of the menopause world, for there are ways to navigate these sartorial minefields with style and grace. Invest in moisture-wicking fabrics that are designed to

Welcome to the Libido Limbo – the chapter where we dive headfirst into the wild and wacky world of menopausal desire, where the ups and downs are as unpredictable as a game of musical chairs at a retirement home. As we navigate this rollercoaster ride of libido fluctuations, let's grab our sense of humor, hold on tight, and see if we can't find some laughs amidst the chaos.

First things first, let's address the elephant in the room – the dreaded "M" word: menopause. It's the hormonal hurricane that can wreak havoc on your desire faster than you can say "hormone replacement therapy." One minute, you're feeling friskier than a spring lamb in heat, and the next, you'd rather cuddle up with a good book and a hot water bottle than engage in any kind of hanky-panky. It's a libido limbo like no other – one where the rules are constantly changing and the stakes couldn't be higher.

But fear not, intrepid traveler of the libido limbo, for you are not alone in your struggles. From hot flashes to mood swings to vaginal dryness that could rival the Sahara desert, menopause throws plenty of obstacles in the path of desire. But with a little creativity, a touch of patience, and a whole lot of laughter, you can navigate this minefield of menopausal libido fluctuations with grace and humor.

Let's start by embracing the humor in the situation. After all, there's something undeniably hilarious about trying to summon your inner sex kitten while simultaneously battling hot flashes and night sweats. It's like trying to light a fire in a rainstorm – sure, it's possible, but it's going to take some serious dedication and a whole lot of perseverance. So why not embrace the absurdity of it all and have a good laugh along the way?

Next, let's talk about communication – the cornerstone of any healthy relationship, especially when it comes to navigating the ups and downs of desire during menopause. It's important to be open and honest with your partner about what you're experiencing – whether it's a sudden surge of desire or a total lack thereof. After all, they can't read your mind, and trying to play guessing games in the bedroom is a recipe for disaster. So grab a glass of wine, sit down with your partner, and have a good old-fashioned heart-to-heart about what's going on between the sheets.

But what about those times when desire feels like it's gone into hibernation, never to return? It's easy to feel discouraged and defeated when you're stuck in the libido limbo, but remember – this too shall pass. Menopause is a temporary phase, and your desire will ebb and flow like the tides of the ocean. So instead of dwelling on what you can't do, focus on what you can – whether it's exploring new ways to connect with your partner, rediscovering the joys of self-pleasure, or simply enjoying the intimacy and closeness that comes from cuddling and snuggling.

Now, let's talk about the importance of self-care in navigating the libido limbo. Taking care of yourself – physically, emotionally, and mentally – is crucial for maintaining a healthy libido during menopause. This might involve prioritizing relaxation techniques like deep breathing or meditation to reduce stress and anxiety, engaging in regular exercise to boost your mood and energy levels, or exploring alternative therapies like acupuncture or massage to enhance your sense of well-being. And don't forget about the power of laughter – whether it's watching a funny movie, reading a humorous book, or sharing a joke with friends, laughter has been shown to improve mood, reduce stress, and even increase libido. So don't be afraid to let loose and have a good chuckle – your libido will thank you for it!

As you navigate the ups and downs of desire in the libido limbo, remember this: you are not defined by your libido, and you are not alone in your struggles. With a sense of humor, a willingness to communicate openly with your partner, and a commitment to self-care, you can navigate the challenges of menopausal desire with grace and humor. So embrace the absurdity, laugh off the obstacles, and remember that the libido limbo is just a temporary phase in the grand adventure of menopause.

Chapter 10: The Partner Predicament: Explaining Menopause to Your Significant Other Without Starting World War III

Welcome to the chapter on "The Partner Predicament" – where we tackle the delicate art of explaining menopause to your significant other without causing chaos, confusion, or the outbreak of World War III. As you embark on this comedic adventure through the minefield of menopausal communication, remember to pack your sense of humor, a healthy dose of patience, and perhaps a few peace offerings to smooth over any potential conflicts.

First things first, let's address the elephant in the room – the fact that menopause isn't exactly a topic that inspires pillow talk. In fact, it's more likely to send your partner running for the hills faster than you can say "hot flash." But fear not, intrepid communicator of the menopause world, for with a little creativity, a touch of humor, and a whole lot of love, you can navigate this conversation with grace and finesse.

Let's start by setting the stage for the conversation. Choose a time when both you and your partner are relaxed, calm, and free from distractions – preferably not right after a heated argument or during a commercial break of their favorite TV show. You want to create an atmosphere of openness and receptivity, where both parties feel comfortable expressing themselves without fear of judgment or misunderstanding.

Next, approach the conversation with honesty and transparency. Be clear about what you're experiencing – whether it's hot flashes, mood swings, or changes in libido – and how it's impacting your day-to-day life. Remember, your partner can't read your mind, so it's important to communicate your needs and feelings openly and honestly. And don't be afraid to inject a little humor into the conversation – after all, laughter is the best medicine, even when it comes to discussing menopause.

But what about those moments when the conversation veers off course and threatens to descend into chaos? It's easy to feel frustrated or overwhelmed when your partner doesn't seem to understand or empathize with what you're going through. But remember, they're navigating uncharted territory too – and they may need a little time and patience to process the information and adjust their perspective. So take a deep breath, count to ten, and try to approach the conversation with compassion and understanding, even when it feels like you're speaking different languages.

Now, let's talk about the importance of education in navigating the partner predicament. Menopause may be a foreign concept to your significant other, but that doesn't mean they can't learn – and it certainly doesn't mean you have to be the sole source of information. Encourage your partner to do their own research, whether it's reading books, watching videos, or attending support groups for partners of menopausal women. The more they understand about what you're going through, the better equipped they'll be to support you and navigate this journey together.

But what if your partner still doesn't seem to get it, despite your best efforts at communication and education? It's easy to feel frustrated or resentful when your needs aren't being met, but remember – it takes two to tango, and navigating the partner predicament is a team effort. Instead of pointing fingers or assigning blame, try to approach the situation with empathy and compassion, and work together to find solutions that meet both of your needs. Whether it's seeking couples counseling, exploring alternative therapies, or simply carving out time for open and honest communication, there are plenty of ways to bridge the gap and strengthen your relationship in the process.

As you navigate the partner predicament and attempt to explain menopause to your significant other without starting World War III, remember this: you are not alone in your struggles, and you don't have to navigate this journey alone. With a sense of humor, a willingness to communicate openly and honestly, and a commitment to education and understanding, you can bridge the gap and strengthen your relationship in the process. So take a deep breath, summon your inner diplomat, and remember that love conquers all – even the challenges of menopause.

Chapter 11: The Beautiful Buffet: Embracing Your Inner Goddess Despite the Wrinkles and Gray Hairs

Welcome to "The Beautiful Buffet" – the chapter where we celebrate the glorious smorgasbord of beauty that comes with embracing your inner goddess, wrinkles, gray hairs, and all. As we navigate the ups and downs of menopause, one thing becomes abundantly clear: beauty is not defined by age, and true radiance comes from within. So grab a plate, load up on self-love, and let's dive into this delicious feast of empowerment and humor.

First things first, let's talk about the elephant in the room – the inevitable changes that come with aging. From wrinkles and gray hairs to sagging skin and everything in between, menopause can feel like a one-way ticket to the land of lost youth. But fear not, dear reader, for with a little perspective and a healthy dose of humor, we can turn these perceived imperfections into badges of honor, proof of a life well-lived and a spirit that refuses to be tamed.

Let's start with wrinkles – those pesky little lines that seem to multiply overnight like rabbits in a vegetable garden. Instead of waging war against these signs of aging, why not embrace them as a testament to your wisdom, experience, and resilience? After all, each wrinkle tells a story – a laugh shared with friends, a tear shed in sorrow, a moment of deep introspection – and together, they form a roadmap of your journey through life. So wear your wrinkles like a badge of honor, and remember that laughter lines are the most beautiful wrinkles of all.

Next, let's tackle gray hairs – those silver strands that seem to sprout up like weeds in a garden of youth. Instead of reaching for the hair dye and trying to turn back the clock, why not embrace your gray hairs as a symbol of your wisdom and maturity? After all, gray hair is just God's way of saying, "Congratulations, you've earned your stripes." So rock those silver locks with pride, and remember that age is just a number – and a little gray hair never hurt anyone.

But what about those other signs of aging – the sagging skin, the age spots, the cellulite that seems to appear overnight like mushrooms after a rainstorm? Instead of lamenting the loss of your youthful appearance, why not celebrate the beauty that comes with embracing your body exactly as it is? After all, beauty is not defined by the size of your waistline or the smoothness of your skin – it's defined by the light that shines from within, the twinkle in your eye, and the laughter that bubbles up from your soul. So love your body, flaws and all, and remember that true beauty comes from embracing your unique essence and letting your light shine bright.

Now, let's talk about the importance of self-care in embracing your inner goddess during menopause. Taking care of yourself – physically, emotionally, and spiritually – is crucial for maintaining your sense of beauty and vitality as you navigate this transformative phase of life. This might involve prioritizing relaxation techniques like yoga or meditation to reduce stress and promote a sense of inner peace, engaging in regular exercise to boost your mood and energy levels, or indulging in pampering rituals like bubble baths or facials to nourish your body and soul. And don't forget about the power of laughter – whether it's sharing a joke with friends, watching a funny movie, or simply finding humor in the absurdities of life, laughter has been shown to improve mood, reduce stress, and increase feelings of well-being. So don't be afraid to let loose and laugh until your sides ache – your inner goddess will thank you for it!

As you embrace your inner goddess and celebrate the beauty of your journey through menopause, remember this: you are a radiant, powerful, and resilient woman, capable of embracing your unique beauty and shining bright at any age. So wear your wrinkles like a crown, rock your gray hairs like a queen, and strut your stuff with confidence and grace. The beautiful buffet of life is yours for the taking – so load up your plate, savor every bite, and remember that true beauty knows no bounds. Cheers to embracing your inner goddess and celebrating the beauty of every stage of life!

Chapter 12: Menopause, Mastery, and Mayhem: Finding Peace, Sanity, and Laughter in the Midst of Hormonal Chaos

Welcome to the grand finale of our menopause journey – a chapter dedicated to finding peace, sanity, and laughter in the midst of hormonal chaos. As we bid adieu to hot flashes, mood swings, and all the other delights of menopause, let's take a moment to reflect on the wild ride we've been on and celebrate the fact that we've survived – with our sense of humor intact and our sanity (mostly) intact.

First things first, let's acknowledge the elephant in the room – menopause is no walk in the park. It's more like a rollercoaster ride through the seven circles of hormonal hell, complete with unexpected twists, stomach-churning drops, and the occasional loop-de-loop. But fear not, dear reader, for with a little humor, a healthy dose of perspective, and perhaps a stiff drink or two, we can navigate this hormonal minefield with grace and laughter.

Let's start by embracing the chaos – after all, laughter is the best medicine, even when it feels like your hormones are staging a full-scale revolt. So grab your sense of humor and prepare to laugh in the face of adversity, because trust me, there will be plenty of opportunities for hilarity along the way. Whether it's mistaking your hot flash for a sudden onset of tropical fever or accidentally using your night sweat as a makeshift hair gel, finding the humor in the madness is key to maintaining your sanity in the midst of hormonal chaos.

Next, let's talk about finding peace amidst the storm. Menopause may be a turbulent time, but it's also an opportunity to cultivate inner peace and resilience in the face of adversity. Whether it's through meditation, mindfulness, or simply taking a few moments each day to breathe deeply and connect with yourself, finding moments of calm amidst the chaos can help you navigate the ups and downs of menopause with grace and ease. And don't forget the power of laughter – there's nothing like a good belly laugh to chase away the stress and bring a little sunshine into even the darkest of days.

But what about finding sanity in the midst of hormonal madness? It's easy to feel like you're losing your mind when your hormones are staging a coup d' tat, but remember – you are not alone in your struggles, and you are not defined by your symptoms. Reach out to friends, family, or a therapist who can provide support and understanding during this challenging time, and don't be afraid to ask for help when you need it. And remember, it's okay to laugh at yourself – after all, sometimes the only way to stay sane in the midst of hormonal chaos is to embrace the madness and laugh until your sides ache.

Finally, let's talk about the importance of finding laughter in the midst of it all. Laughter is not only a powerful coping mechanism, but it's also a source of strength, resilience, and joy in the face of adversity. So don't be afraid to embrace the absurdity of menopause, to laugh at the ridiculousness of hot flashes and mood swings, and to find humor in the most unexpected of places. After all, life is too short to take it too seriously – so grab your sense of humor and prepare to laugh your way through menopause, one hot flash at a time.

As we bid farewell to menopause, let's raise a glass to the laughter, the tears, and the moments of sheer madness that have defined this wild and wacky journey. May we emerge on the other side stronger, wiser, and more fabulous than ever before – armed with a sense of humor, a touch of grace, and the knowledge that we can conquer anything life throws our way, even the seven circles of hormonal hell. Here's to menopause, mastery, and mayhem – may we laugh in the face of chaos and emerge victorious on the other side. Cheers!